MALE ENHANCEMENT

YOUR OPTIONS TO PENIS ENLARGEMENT

PENIS SURGERY, PENIS STRETCHERS, PENIS PUMPS, PENIS CLAMPS, PENIS PILLS, AND PENIS EXERCISE

Richard Nelson

Table of Contents

The follow book is reproduced below with the goal of providing information that is as accurate and reliable as possible. Regardless, purchasing this book can be seen as consent to the fact that both the publisher and the author of this book are in no way experts on the topics discussed within and that any recommendations or suggestions that are made herein are for entertainment purposes only. Professionals should be consulted as needed prior to undertaking any of the action endorsed herein.

This declaration is deemed fair and valid by both the American Bar Association and the Committee of Publishers Association and is legally binding throughout the United States.

Furthermore, the transmission, duplication or reproduction of any of the following work including specific information will be considered an illegal act irrespective of if it is done electronically or in print. This extends to creating a secondary or tertiary copy of the work or a recorded copy and is only allowed with express written consent from the Publisher. All additional right reserved.

The information in the following pages is broadly considered to be a truthful and accurate account of facts and as such any inattention, use or misuse of the information in question by the reader will render any resulting actions solely under their purview. There are no scenarios in which the publisher or the original author of this work can be in any fashion deemed liable for any hardship or damages that may befall them after undertaking information described herein.

Additionally, the information in the following pages is intended only for informational purposes and should thus be thought of as universal. As befitting its nature, it is presented without assurance regarding its prolonged validity or interim quality. Trademarks that are mentioned are done without written consent and can in no way be considered an endorsement from the trademark holder.

INTRODUCTION

Congratulations on downloading *Penis Enlargement Options* and thank you for doing so.

The male sex organ plays an important role in our lives, our society, and our culture. It has been the focus of psychology, of satire, and even philosophy. Figures from literature all the way back to the ancient Greeks have chimed in with their opinions.

Sophocles, one of the great Grecian tragic poets once said that "having one is like being chained to a madman," something just about every man has realized at least once or twice in his life.

This book makes an assumption, namely that the reader is looking to improve his sex life and feels increasing the size of his penis will be the answer. In truth, while it is possible to increase the length and girth of your member, the resulting improvement will be noticeable, but not spectacular. You may also even be surprised to learn that most women do not have a "bigger is better" philosophy.

Of course, there is more to a good sex life than just size. As men get older, performance expectations suffer somewhat as just another cost of aging. When you consider the effects of a sedentary, fast food lifestyle, then even more reasons for poor performance and perceived inadequacy come into play.

The following chapters will discuss how you can improve the size and performance of your penis and improve your sex life. While there are no "miracles" when it comes to male enhancement, there are a variety of tools, supplements, exercise, and lifestyle changes that can lead to a significant improvement.

You may have noticed, there are a lot of products out there aimed at men who want to improve their penis size and thickness. A search of the Amazon web site using just the word "penis," returned more than 34,000 products, some of which were truly disturbing. Combine "penis" and "sexual wellness," and you get even more choices (nearly 46,000). It would seem a lot of men have found a need for assistance in the bedroom (and based on some of the products, there are a good number of single women who have searched for temporary (?) substitutes for male companionship.

In fact, during the course of researching this book, I found lots of web sites offering information on the subject of penis enlargement and erectile dysfunction. What was surprising was how little actual information there was to be found. All those web pages were basically expounding on the same few things. Much of it was advertising, filled with lots of wonderful claims, but backed by very little proof or scientific information. Over the counter supplements were plentiful, and their claims bordered on the magical.

I also picked up some interesting information regarding our little buddy. For instance, did you know that in the womb, we all start out with a clitoris? It isn't until hormones start pumping that the male sex organ starts forming.

Even more interesting, and perhaps a little bit frightening, is the fact that you can actually break your penis (ouch!). One thing that makes this so interesting is that even though we often refer to the erection as a "boner," there is no bone in the human penis. A broken penis usually occurs when an accident happens while a man is erect. Fortunately, the treatment is fairly simple, if inconvenient; six weeks on bed while wearing a penis splint.

And there is also one other bit of good news for the human male. As far as primates go, we're the biggest. By comparison, an adult gorilla, fully erect only reaches about an inch and a half on average. So in actually, that old cliché about someone "being hung like a gorilla" is more insult than compliment.

Most of the science there is on this topic has been focused on "boner pills" rather than penis enlargement. There is also a thriving sex toy industry that is perfectly happy selling and promoting products designed to make you bigger, harder, and longer lasting. You can also "accessorize" your member in all sorts of ways, some silly, some romantic, some kinky, and some just plain weird.

So how do you wade through all the crap?

This book will help you. It will educate you on the many different options out there and provide information as to their effectiveness and risks. It doesn't promise you a miracle, but I'm sure you'll find improvement here.

You'll also get more information on erectile dysfunction and ways of dealing with it. Erectile dysfunction can go hand in hand with penis size, and more than 30 million men in the United States are dealing with this issue. If a man is over 40 years old, there is a 50 percent chance he has this problem.

Make a web search using the words "penis enlargement," or "erectile dysfunction," and you will find thousands of web pages offering all sorts of "cures." These "cures" are often a combination of herbs and other "natural" ingredients and promise the impossible.

If they were harmless, it wouldn't be much of a problem. You have more than likely heard of the "placebo" effect. This is where the patient is given a pill and told it is a drug to cure their affliction. In spite of the "drug" being little more than a sugar pill, patients responded as if the drug was real.

In reality, some of these over the counter supplements can cause more problems than they solve.

There are plenty of books on this subject on the market, thanks again for choosing this one! Every effort was made to ensure it is full of as much useful information as possible, please enjoy!

CHAPTER 1: DOES SIZE MATTER?

This is not an unusual question. What may surprise you though is that men and women tend to answer the question differently. Men, perhaps not surprisingly, tend to worry more about penis size than women do.

While it may not seem that way in the world of pornography, where men sport boners that could be used to provide shade for a small village, and women often display breasts that could do the same, as usual, in the real world, it's different.

The truth is the average or "normal" woman has limits to the size of the penis she is willing to accommodate. A super huge member is painful and uncomfortable, and really doesn't make any improvement in the quality of their sexual pleasure. In fact, it can do just the opposite. It can hurt instead of please.

Now that I've gotten that out of the way, the idea that a man is reading this book in hopes of improving the quality of his and his partner's sexual experiences is a positive. There's nothing wrong at all with wanting to be a better performer and being willing to make such an effort is the sign of a dedicated lover.

By the way, it is certainly possible to effect some changes in the length and girth of your penis. You won't work miracles and you wont necessarily see fast results, but they will help you improve. They can also help with your performance in general.

Some other good news is that a few of these methods are low cost, easy to use, may spice up your sex life, and are temporary. Believe it or not, temporary can be good. It gives you options. It may surprise you, but women don't necessarily find that bigger is "better." How frustrating would it be to actually increase your size and then find out the object of your affection no longer wants to have sex with you because you're "too big?"

WHAT IS NORMAL?

The average penis length is a little more than 5 inches when erect and about 4.6 inches in diameter, also while erect. In fact, if yours is between 4 inches and 6.3 inches when erect, you fit in with 90 percent of all men according to a review of 17 different studies that evaluated more than 15,000 men. In fact, a flaccid penis needs to be shorter than 1.6 inches long to be considered short by medical science.

So what about all those giant "tools" you see in porn? Well, I'm sure a few are freaks of nature, while others are "enhanced" via computer wizardry. It is also possible that in a few cases, steroids may have been involved, although I haven't found anything to indicate that there are steroids that work that way.

This doesn't mean you should give up your goals of improved performance. It does mean you shouldn't feel threatened because your "best buddy" doesn't enter the room a few minutes before you do.

What do Women Think About Penis Size?

This may come as a surprise to you, but size isn't very high on the typical woman's radar. Surveys and interviews repeatedly show women are really quite happy with "average" and a bit put off by "huge" because it hurts.

Most women (there are always outliers) are more concerned with how well the man uses his "rod" than they are how long it is. In fact, one of the few respondents who did think a bigger penis was better thought that because "I think bigger men are more confident and that makes them better in bed," she said.

So even for her, it was the guy's confidence that was important, and not so much his size.

WELL, WHAT ABOUT VAGINA SIZE?

Good question. If we're worried about penis length, doesn't it make sense to consider the "receptacle?"

As it happens, the human vagina is a difficult thing to measure. Think about it, on one hand, a tampon can fill one, but on the other hand, a baby can fit through it. (WebMd).

Masters and Johnson, the sex researchers from the 1960s, actually measured 100 women's vaginas (how would you like to be able to put "vagina measurer" on your resume?), both stimulated and unstimulated according to WebMd.

They found that unstimulated, the average vagina measured from 2.75 to 3.25 inches. Stimulated, they increased in size to a range from 4.25 to 4.75 inches. Hmm... kind of sounds like nature had a plan here doesn't it? The average penis seems to fit the average vagina pretty well doesn't it?

So What's All the Fuss About?

Physical conditions, health concerns, and other issues can affect the penis and its size. A man can have an average or even longer than average penis, but not show it because he is overweight (the shaft sinks into the fat making the penis appear shorter) or may have trouble getting or maintaining an erection.

Oh yeah, it also seems the most sensitive part of the vagina is the outer third, adding credence to the old saying "it's not the length, it's what you do with it." Too long, and it appears all you're really doing is jostling the groceries digesting in the stomach. Many women have said they do not find this to be a pleasurable sensation. You may also want to remember the woman's "G" spot is located in the upper wall of the vagina about a third of the way in.

Okay. That's enough of telling you that you don't have a problem. That isn't why you're reading this book, and it isn't why I'm writing it either. In the next chapter we'll start looking at ways to help the "little guy" (sorry) do a better job of reaching his full potential.

For some men, a single pill is enough to do the trick, for others, it may seem like nothing helps. If you fall into the latter category, then consider combining some of the things you learn about in this book. Keep in mind, you should be very careful about mixing over the counter supplements and prescription drugs. Make sure you talk to your doctor before doing so, particularly if you are not in the best of health. A safer approach is mixing a prescribed medication with some of the health suggestions you will learn about and also using some of the devices discussed in this book. You can also try some of the penis exercises as well.

Chapter 2: Prescription Penis Pills Like Viagra and Cialis

Unless you've spent the last few years at the South Pole (and they have internet access at Amundsen Scott South Pole Station, as well as sex), you'll know that medical science has come up with a number of drugs designed to perk up your "Longfellow."

While the big three oral drugs, Viagra, Levitra and Cialis, get most of the advertising time, there are other options. In this chapter you will learn about the prescription drugs that can help you achieve better "personal growth." You will also get a rundown on all of your prescription solutions. These drugs work very well for many men and have been featured in numerous television comedies and other programs.

There are, in fact, some 20 erectile dysfunction drugs that have been approved by the FDA. This includes the generic forms of the three drugs listed above. It also includes drugs that are delivered other ways besides orally. And, there are more being developed every day. You'll learn about them too in this chapter.

Many of these drugs work by increasing blood flow to the penis. This is an important part of establishing and maintaining an erection. There are two larger chambers in the penis shaft. During an erection, these chambers fill with blood, causing the penis to "inflate" and get hard. For most men, the cause of poor erections is insufficient blood flow to the penis. For some though, an accident may have damaged the penis. There are a few other options that can help them.

One final note you should also be aware of. These drugs are also a bit pricey. While many health insurance plans cover the cost of them (with a copay of course), if you don't have health insurance, the cost of sex can become painful for your wallet.

Viagra

Viagra (Sildenafil) was the first of the big name heavily promoted erectile dysfunction drugs. It's generally considered to be an effective medication best taken on an empty stomach about an hour before sex.

Erections are caused by blood flow increasing to the penis and filling two large chambers inside it. Erectile dysfunction is often caused by reduced blood flow to the same place. Viagra works by increasing blood flow to the penis. This by the way, is why blood pressure medications inhibit erections, they lower blood pressure, which reduces blood flow to the penis. It is also why side effects of the drug include flushed skin (more blood saturation), headaches and stuffiness (increased blood flow engorging more than just your penis).

This is generally considered a pretty safe drug unless you're taking a nitrate drug for a heart condition (nitroglycerin is one example) or certain recreational drugs such as "poppers," (amyl nitrate) according to drugs.com.

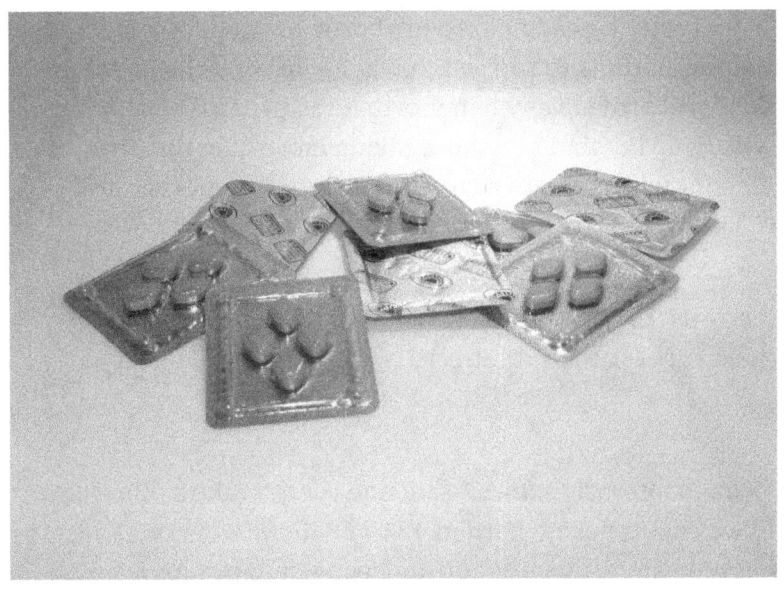

Viagra does also have some potential side effects. Some of these such as sinus pressure are common and pass after a reasonable period of time. Others, such as a decrease to blood pressure in the optic nerve leading to vision loss are more significant, although fortunately not that common.

You still need sexual stimulation for an erection even with Viagra. Also, it is possible to overdose on this drug, and there are some well publicized stories of people doing just that. One such story tells about a Russian user who died after overdosing on the drug during a marathon sex session (apparently he had taken a full bottle of the pills even though there is nothing to suggest that going beyond the prescribed dose will provide any benefits that the prescribed amounts will. Keep in mind too, those taking more than the prescribed amount will also experience amped up side effects too.

Many users report satisfaction with the drug, even if they don't care for the side effects.

"I am in my early sixties," said one user. "I take a 50mg and like clockwork I am hard in 45 to 60 minutes. No worries about keeping the erection long enough to climax. I can't believe just how good this drug works. Side effects for me are minimal."

CIALIS

Another heavily promoted erectile dysfunction drug is Cialis (Tadalafil). Cialis relaxes muscles found in the wall of the blood vessels in the penis and also increases blood flow to it (drugs.com), but is a different type of drug than Viagra. In fact, Cialis is often used to treat BPH (Benign Prostrate

Hyperplasia), something else that makes getting an erection more difficult.

Side effects can include: headache, stomach discomfit, back pain, muscle pain, stuffy nose, flushing, or dizziness according to webmd.com. Users generally experience just one, maybe two of these side effects, not all at once. Most of these side effects pass after the drug's effects wear off, but users are cautioned that if any of the symptoms do persist, they should see their doctor. Many of the same advisories for Viagra also apply to Cialis.

It is possible to overdose on this drug too. Users are cautioned not to exceed their prescribed dose. The FDA limits dosages to 20 mg and normally 2.5 mg is prescribed for an initial dose. Cialis is normally taken only once a day. In fact, one of its selling points is that it doesn't need to be taken precisely an hour before hand like Viagra. It can provide erection help for as long as 36 hours after taking it. It is also not necessary to take it daily unless you plan on having sex on a daily basis (you lucky devil you).

It is also recommended to avoid drinking alcohol or grapefruit juice while on Cialis and also to avoid eating

27

grapefruit. (Of course over consumption of alcohol is another factor in erectile dysfunction, so abstaining from or reducing consumption of alcohol will also help your erection prospects).

Users report generally good results with this drug, although experiences were varied.

"I've had a erection problem for about 7 years. I've always had high Cholesterol; I have had trouble getting a rock hard erection," said one review. "Now I've been on Tadalafil 25ml for a week now. What a difference that has made I'm being woken up with a rock hard erection, what a life saver this is."

Levitra, Staxyn

Levitra and Staxyn are both forms of Vardenafil. This is another drug that works by increasing blood flow to the penis. It generally takes about 30 minutes to work and its effects usually last about 5 hours.

An interesting warning comes with this drug. Users are advised not to eat grapefruit or drink grapefruit juice while using Levitra, since it can increase the risk of side effects. Levitra's side effects tend to be similar to those of Viagra and Cialis. The main reason for this is likely the increased blood flow, which affects blood flow throughout the body and not just the penis.

There are also the same cautions for Levitra as there are for Viagra and Cialis. In addition, people who are taking Alpha Blocker drugs to treat BPH or high blood pressure need to discuss Levitra use with their doctor since the combination of the drugs can cause blood pressure drops that can be serious.

It is possible to overdose from Levitra just as it is possible to overdose from Viagra and Cialis.

Users have generally been happy with their results from this drug. And like the other erectile dysfunction drugs, they can get expensive, particularly if not covered by your insurance plan.

"I am 57 and have tried all the popular ED meds, having low T makes getting and keeping and erection a problem but I personally like Levitra 20 mg, can get rock hard within 20 or 30 minutes of taking it and it's good for several hours afterwards," one reviewer said, "had three orgasms within an 6-7 hour time frame which is about what I could do at age 20, so impressive. Mild headache, flushing and nausea but not bad. Viagra gave me similar results but not as effective for a long as the Levitra. Cialis is a no go for me. Bad leg cramps."

Stendra (Avanafil)

Stendra is another one of the "little blue pill" drugs used to treat erectile dysfunction. It also works by relaxing the blood vessels, much as the other drugs do.

It should be taken no more than once a day. It is usually taken about 30 minutes before sexual activity. (It seems at least a few of these drugs are nature's way of saying "increase your foreplay.")

Users generally began with a 100 mg dose. After that, dosages can range from 50 mg to 200 mg. user reviews on this drug were a bit mixed. Here's one of the positive ones:

"Got off of Cialis because of constant heart burn and read about Stendra and its super fast time to erections," he said. "So got a prescription and started with 200mg. First attempt was amazing and in 30 minutes I was rock hard, just the thought of being able to enter my wife and not cum immediately because I was so stressed about being hard enough to get inside. My wife reported I felt nice and hard and we had great sex. On subsequent times I would say it was 80 percent effective sometimes I would have no problems getting hard, other times manual stimulation was required before I could get inside. Other times I would be inside but I would go soft inside her. "

ERECTILE DYSFUNCTION DRUGS THAT CAN BE INJECTED

I'm not sure whose idea this was, but there is a class of erectile dysfunction drugs that are delivered via injection into the penis. The only silver lining to this is that your doctor can teach you how to do the injections so you can administer the drug in the "comfort" of your own home instead of scheduling a doctor's visit every time you plan on getting "lucky." (Somehow the words "lucky" and "injection into the penis" don't seem like they belong in the same sentence).

Not surprisingly, men who use this drug do report some pain (imagine my surprise) from the injections and also from the high costs of the drug and syringes. The good news is that they also report that the drug used this way is pretty effective, so long as it is properly mixed and injected. Sometimes doctors will prescribe the injectable version with the oral version for particularly "hard" cases (sorry for the bad pun). This of course makes getting an erection even more expensive, since none of the erectile dysfunction drugs can be called cheap.

Injectable medications can help you get an erection when pills can't, which is one of the reasons why they are still prescribed even though they are a bit more complicated. They should not be used more than three times a week.

ALPROSTADIL

This drug can be injected or used as a urethral application (explained in the next section). It works by expanding the blood vessels and increasing blood flow in the penis. The injectable version is sold under the names: "Caverject," "Prostin," and "Edex." Each of these requires a doctor's prescription.

The injectable version tends to be successful for four fifths of the men who use it. It generally takes about five to 20 minutes for it to take effect and its effects are reported to last about an hour and sometimes continue after ejaculation.

There are a variety of risks associated with this drug that are similar to ones with the previously mentioned ones. The approach does offer one risk that isn't associated with the pills, and that is the possibility of a needle breaking off in the penis. (I would imagine this is probably just as bad as it sounds.)

Just like many of the other medicines in this section, you should not drink alcoholic beverages while using it. Elderly users need to be aware that they will often be more sensitive to the drug's effects than younger users.

People who use this medicine report good results with it. One user said: "Very dependable - works every time once you learn how to inject properly. Results start after 15 minutes and last up to almost 2 hours for me. My wife and I love it!"

Urethral Medicines

This next group also relies on the direct method of delivering a drug, but without the pain of a needle. Urethral medicine users insert a dose directly into the penis much like a tiny suppository (with the help of a preloaded plastic tube device). The dose is about half the size of a grain of rice. As you might expect, the experience is not pleasurable. Some users have complained that the drug didn't work very well this way and coupled with the pain from insertion, led to a disappointing sexual experience. Side effects from this drug generally involve localized pain (sure sounds like a mood breaker when you consider where that "localized" pain will occur). In addition, it is possible for an erection that can last from four to six hours. If this happens to you, you should contact your doctor.

Of the three delivery forms, this method generally produces the poorest results.

ALPROSTADIL

As mentioned in the last section, there is a suppository form of this drug (known as "MUSE," an abbreviation for "Medicated Urethral System for Erection). It isn't considered as reliable as the injectable form, and seems to only help about 30 percent to 40 percent of the men who use it. The suppository form has the same side effects as the injectable form.

"After nerve sparing prostate surgery I was prescribed several of the big name drugs but no satisfaction and too many side effects for me," said one user. "My doctor then prescribed Muse (1000mg) a good erection was obtainable nothing like before the surgery but at least it works, as others have suggest standing up sure makes it work faster and last longer, suggest it be used well before expiry date and its extremely important that the application instructions be followed exactly."

IN THE PIPELINE

It probably shouldn't come to anyone as a surprise that medical science is working on additional solutions to the erectile dysfunction problem. It's not safe to say there is a miracle drug just around the corner though. Here's a look at what is coming:

- Uprima (apomorphine) – works by stimulating dopamine, the brain chemical that fires up sexual interest and arousal. It is taken by placing under the tongue where is dissolves. Its side effects include nausea and vomiting (talk about mood killers) and several people have passed out after taking the drug (no word on whether or not they were smiling at the time). While it is currently available in Europe, its release is on hold here in the United States.

- Topiglan (alprostadil) – this is a cream version of the drug described earlier that is injected into the penis or inserted into the penis as a suppository. This isn't as far along the release process as Uprima and hasn't come up for approval yet. It is not even sure how it will be used in treatment and whether it will be combined with injections or penile suppositories.

- Melanocortin activators: these drugs are also early in the pipeline. It appears they may work on the central nervous system via intranasal application (via the nose). It also seems these drugs only work for patients dealing with psychological or emotional issues that hinder erections. They do not appear to offer any help to those with medically caused erectile dysfunction.

- Gene therapy – designed to provide proteins that are missing in the penis to help improve erections. As you might imagine, this one will take a long time to get approved.

CHAPTER 3: OVER THE COUNTER PILLS AND HERBS

If you've watched late night TV or spent any time on the Internet, you've seen ads for supplements or pills that will "guarantee" an erection or a bigger penis. Some of these may actually have ingredients that are believed to help somewhat, while others are merely "hopeful." An important consideration for anyone considering taking one of these supplements is that they are not nearly as heavily scrutinized as FDA approved medicines and their labels aren't always accurate either. There's a reason doctors have to prescribe certain drugs, the best medical science says there are potential harms in those drugs even though they provide a benefit. The knowledge of a medical professional is deemed to be necessary to avoid tragedy.

The fact that over the counter supplements do not require a prescription or a doctor's advice is not necessarily a good thing, particularly if you have pre-existing medical conditions or are taking prescription medications. If either of these are true in your case, talk to your doctor before taking such supplements.

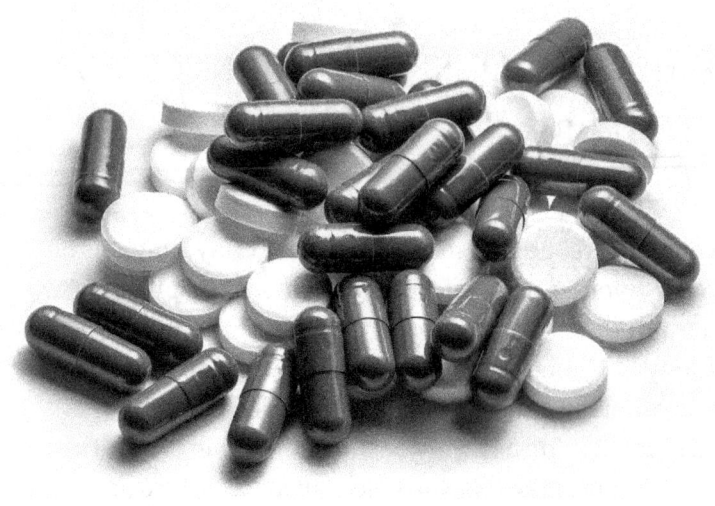

The Mayo Clinic has identified four herbal remedies in particular that show some promise in clinical studies. These four are DHEA, L-arginine, Ginseng, and Yohimbe. We'll look at these and a variety of other options.

Keep in mind, "show some promise," is not exactly a ringing endorsement. Still, the clinical research process is often conservative in its assessments. There can be any number of reasons why researchers are cautious about assessing results. The study sample size may be too small to establish much confidence, or it may not be possible to exclude other factors that can play a role in the study's findings. These are just a couple of reasons for the caution that researchers show when evaluating study results.

As one doctor said, there is a bit of the "placebo effect" with these supplements. Sometimes just telling someone a product works will help them achieve the desired results even though the product actually does nothing. This makes it hard for researchers to be sure the effects they are seeing are from the product being tested. Another caution, when supplements do work, the process is usually cumulative. In other words, you need to take them for a while to see the effects.

Still, let's take a closer look at these four along with some other supplements that are reputed to provide some aid with erections and improving penis size. Also, if you do decide to go with supplements, it is often best to go with ones where the specific ingredient you are looking for is the only ingredient in the supplement (a binding agent to hold the pill together is probably okay).

DHEA

Dehydroepiandrosterone, otherwise known as "DHEA," has shown some ability to increase sexual desire in women and some help with erectile dysfunction in men. It also appears to be safe in low doses.

According to WebMd.com, the reason DHEA may offer some help to erectile dysfunction sufferers is because it is the hormone the human body converts into testosterone. If your body is not producing enough of this hormone, DHEA can make a difference. If it is, then taking this supplement won't make a difference. Since low testosterone can be a cause of erectile dysfunction, improving your body's production of it can improve your erections.

If you do start taking DHEA, be aware that increased acne is a potential side effect. Also, trying to find the right dose can be confusing. At the Mayo Clinic's web site, several different doses and dosing patterns are listed. The smallest was 20-75 mg by mouth for six months, but there is also a single 300 mg dosage, and several other versions involving greater dosages.

Considering the uncertainty, it may certainly be worth a conversation with your doctor before starting a DHEA regimen, particularly if you have other health issues. Since DHEA seems to have negative reactions with a wide variety of medications, discussing it with your doctor before starting taking it should be considered very important.

L-ARGININE

This amino acid is found in many of the foods we eat, including red meat, poultry, fish, and dairy products. It is a popular supplement with many uses including treating erectile dysfunction.

Like many erectile dysfunction approaches, it works by opening up blood vessels for improved blood flow. This happens when the body converts the amino acid to nitric oxide.

If you have high blood pressure or a heart condition calling for the use of nitroglycerin or other similar medications, talk to your doctor before using L-arginine since it also lowers blood pressure. It may also cause blood pressure problems if taken with Viagra since that also lowers blood pressure.

The recommended dose for erectile dysfunction is five grams a day. Some products pair this amino acid up with pycnogenol, and they do seem to work well together.

Ginseng

It can help, nobody knows why, but at least it won't do much harm. Not exactly a ringing endorsement, but at least it's safe. Red ginseng (also known as "Asian" ginseng) appears to work better. Keep in mind it can also increase the effects of caffeine in the body (not a complaint for some of us) and also interfere with the effects of some medications (meaning you should talk to your doctor before trying it if you are taking prescription medications).

It is the root of the Ginseng plant that is used for these supplements. To be effective, the root must be at least five years old. This means good quality Ginseng supplements will be more expensive than poor quality ones (I know that sounds obvious, but it isn't always the case).

YOHIMBE

Yohimbe is made from the bark of an African tree and has been shown to help with erectile dysfunction. It also has been shown to have a lot of side effects. You definitely want a doctor involved with any decision to try this one.

There is also a drug with a similar sounding name, "yohimbine hydrochloride," that has used to treat erectile dysfunction for decades. This is not the same thing as Yohimbe, and it requires a prescription. Yohimbe is not a substitute for the prescription drug either.

PROPIONYL-L-CARNITINE

If you're taking Viagra, then this supplement may be worth considering according to the Mayo Clinic web site. It says that some studies have shown that taking Propionyl L carnitine combined with Viagra may show better results than using Viagra alone. You should check with your doctor before trying this though.

GINKGO BILOBA

Ginkgo Biloba is one of those things that is promoted for all sorts of "magical" health properties, including perking up the penis. While it can help with blood flow, it is not helpful with erectile dysfunction, according to Eric Laborde, MD, a spokesman for the American Urological Association.

YOHIMBINE (HYDROCHLORIDE)

This is only available via a doctor's prescription. Yohimbine (hydrochloride) is used to increase blood flow. It has been found to increase erections, but takes from two to three weeks to work. There are a number of potential side effects and potential drug interaction problems with this medicine, which is why it is only available via prescription. It is important that you coordinate its use with a doctor. This includes follow up consultations so long as you are using it.

Melatonin II

This is not the same as melatonin, which has not been shown to help with erectile dysfunction. While this lab made hormone substitute has shown some promise with erectile dysfunction, it also needs to be injected into the penis. If you're going to going to that much trouble, you are probably better off with one of the prescription injectable drugs instead.

L-citrulline

This is another amino acid that helps with erectile dysfunction by helping the body make more arginine, which helps it produce more nitric oxide. Some doctors recommend it over L-arginine, since that amino acid tends to require large doses to do anything helpful. High doses of this supplement can also lower your blood pressure, so if you're on drugs for high blood pressure, you may want to discuss this one with your doctor before giving it a try. The general recommendation is 500 to 1,000 mg. Combining this supplement with Arginine is generally considered a good idea, and Citrulline can also be used with other penile enhancement substitutes. Most experts will tell you it's better to get this from the food you eat rather than through a supplement.

HORNY GOAT WEED (EPIMEDIUM)

As you might guess, an American marketing firm did not name this product. It is in fact, a traditional Chinese approach to improve penis size and erections. When you consider how populous the country is, it is certainly understandable that American consumers have put their faith in it. Supposedly, the herb has been used in Asian countries for some 2,000 years as an aphrodisiac and to help with sexual dysfunction. There have not been any clinical studies confirming this though.

It has been tested on rats, with good results too (just what we need, more rats), but it has not been tested on humans. It does seem to boost energy, but it can also lower blood pressure. The herb works in a way similar to that of Viagra, but it isn't as potent. There is no standardized dose, and it probably won't work as quickly as the prescription drug either.

There is a substance in the herb that helps block an enzyme which restricts blood flow to the penis (maybe those Chinese goats knew something after all) according to a 2008 study (WebMD) and may in fact, be a reasonable alternative to prescription erectile dysfunction drugs. The study should not be considered definitive though. Still, it is available over the counter and does not appear to have many of the side effects the prescription drugs do. It also does have some side effects and long term use is not recommended.

USA Supplement's Horny Goat weed with Maca is a popular version of this traditional Chinese herb. You can find it via this link: Horny Goat Weed. Many people I have encountered have had good natural results by using horny goat weed, and I have had clients who have seen good results with the product Mr. Thick , Male Enhancement. You can find it available on Amazon.com.

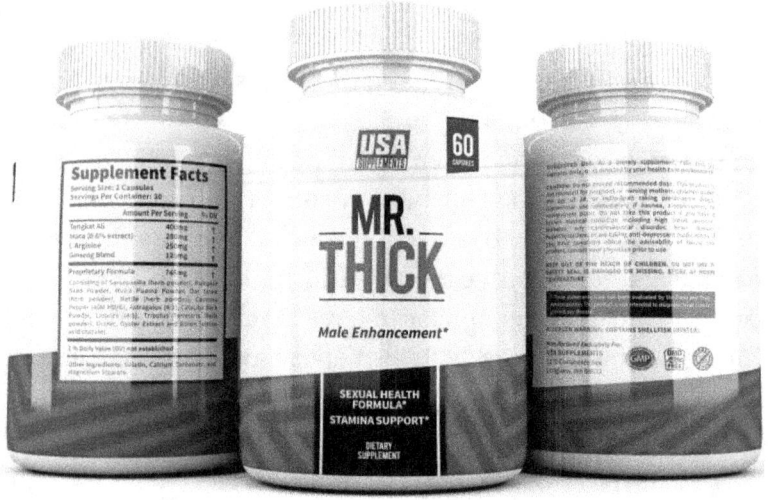

Zinc

If you have a zinc deficiency it may be playing a roll in your erectile dysfunction. According to WebMD, low testosterone and zinc deficiency may be related, so taking zinc may help you if you have such a deficiency. Even if it doesn't help your sexual performance, zinc is generally credited with being effective at preventing colds, and in moderate doses, appears very safe to take. Adding a zinc supplement to your daily routine appears to have a pretty good upside, with minimal downside.

CREATINE

There are several benefits to taking this supplement including increasing cell energy and improving muscle recovery time. It also affects smooth muscle growth (there are smooth muscle areas in the penis), so it can help with penis enlargement. Two to three grams a day is considered sufficient. People who are physically active tend to do better with Creatine than those who don't. This substance is banned in many pro sports, so if you are an athlete (NCAA or pro), you should probably check with the appropriate specialists to make sure you're not breaking any rules by taking this supplement.

FLAVONOIDS

Studies have shown that men who eat a diet heavy with flavonoids, are less likely to have erectile dysfunction. This doesn't mean they can prevent it though. It just shows a correlation (when one thing happens, the other thing tends to occur), and not that flavonoids prevent erectile dysfunction.

Fortunately, lots of foods contain flavonoids. These include berries, tree fruits, vegetables, and spices. Juices made from whole fruits, red wine, and many teas also contain flavonoids.

VITAMIN D

If your erectile dysfunction was caused by an accident, then Vitamin D may be helpful. One study has shown that many men with erectile dysfunction also have Vitamin D deficiencies.

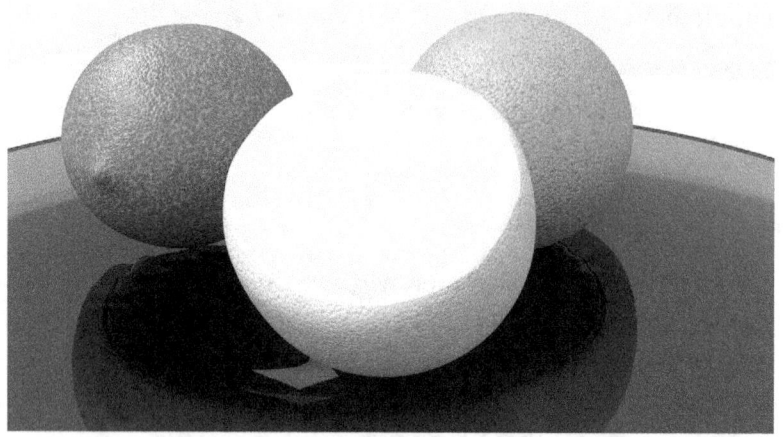

DAMIANA

This is one of those "wonder" herbs that is claimed to do everything but clean the kitchen sink. Some of the claims for it including improving mental function, treating, headache, depression, upset stomach, constipation, improve sexual function, and others.

There is no medical evidence to support any of these claims. Damiana is known to affect blood sugar levels, so if you are a diabetic and plan on taking it, be sure to monitor your blood sugar carefully.

ACCUPUNCTURE

Okay. This is not an over the counter medication, but it certainly can be thought of as an alternative treatment approach. Unfortunately, there is really no evidence it can do anything to help. Any success stories associated with this form of treatment are probably more likely a result of the placebo effect.

CREAMS

There are a variety of creams that claim to improve your erection and perhaps plump up your "Johnson" or prolong your erection. Ingredients vary and there really isn't much in the way of regulation of these products, so check the labels carefully. Many contain benzocaine, a numbing agent, so you can expect reduced sensations. This is probably what helps delay ejaculation, but may also reduce your enjoyment of the experience.

TONG BALM

This is advertised as an old Chinese herbal remedy. It is a type of balm (cream). The user takes a very small dab and applies it to the underside of the head of the penis right where it connects to the shaft. Some instructions say to apply once an hour for three hours before sex, but many users say once is enough.

One of the attractions to this product is that it supposedly heightens sensations rather than numbing them. It is also supposed to provide better control over ejaculation helping the user prolong sex. Tong Balm usually comes in very small amounts, which goes with the recommendation to only use a little at a time.

PENIS PATCHES

If you have ever tried to quit smoking using a nicotine patch, you know that as far as drug delivery systems go, applying a patch to your skin is not particularly difficult.

It is now possible to find patches that release herbal erectile dysfunction remedies. Because the herbal release occurs slowly and over a greater period of time than the same herbal concoction, its effects (if any) should last longer.

Penis patches can be placed anywhere on the body (and probably shouldn't be placed on the penis itself) and can take a few days to produce results. They also tend to be more expensive than their herbal supplement counterparts. Some patch makers stress combining their product with an exercise program.

CHAPTER 4: EXERCISES AND DEVICES

If you're more of a "hands on" kind of guy (sorry about the pun), then exercises and or accessories can be just what you need. While you still can't expect miracles, improvement in length and girth are possible.

Since there is muscle in the penis, the idea that exercising it (not the way you think) might lead to an increase in size isn't an unreasonable supposition. The exercises work along the idea that most exercises do, you're trying to break down existing muscle tissue and build it back up.

Simply put, there are two separate exercise purposes. One group of exercises works on stretching the ligaments of the penis to make it longer. The other group of exercises focuses on increasing the blood capacity of the penis making its girth bigger.

Just a word of warning, these are definitely hands on, and not for your workout at the gym. And a warm, damp towel will aid in comfort and stretching.

STRETCHING EXERCISES

These involve stretching your penis in different ways and different directions. Unlike the stretching exercises you do to warm up for a regular workout, these stretching exercises are said to actually help you increase the length of your "Johnson."

While it takes time for these exercises to show an improvement, you'll at least be able to keep track of your progress by occasionally measuring your penis both while flaccid and erect. Another nice thing about this approach is that it doesn't cost you anything. One challenge though is that for many people is the time commitment involved. In order to achieve measurable results, it is necessary to devote about a half hour a day, four to five days a week for a number of months. Many people just do not have that kind of private time to devote to this kind of exercise program.

There is a word of warning for you though. Don't fall for the old athlete's mantra, "No pain, no gain." These exercises shouldn't be very painful. If your best buddy hurts while your stretching it, then it likely means you are exerting too much force.

For some of these exercises you might find some kind of skin friendly lubricant helpful. For others, a warm towel might be a better choice.

Let's start with the most basic exercises:

THE CIRCLE JERK

Okay, that's not really what it's called. And there is definitely no jerking involved. Start by making a circle with your thumb and forefinger (yes, an "Okay" sign). Position the circle right on the shaft of your penis, just below its head.

There are five stretches in this exercise, one in each direction. You're going to stretch your penis Up, Down, Left,

Right, and Straight out there. Make your stretches slow and steady and back off if it starts to become painful. You can be standing or sitting when you do this, but the exercise should only be done with a flaccid penis.

JELQING

Fortunately, this exercise is easier to do than it is to pronounce. Let's start by forming the same finger grip that we used for the last exercise. Instead of placing it below the head of the penis, start with at the base of the shaft. Now, using light pressure, slowly move your hand up the shaft. You should feel your shaft being stretched. If you don't, then your grip can be a little bit tighter, but once again, pain means you're trying to hard.

The idea behind Jelqing is that it helps move blood to the head of the penis. The good news is that it is pretty safe so long as you don't overdo it. The bad news is there isn't a lot of evidence to suggest that it works. In fact, most medical professionals say it won't do you any good.

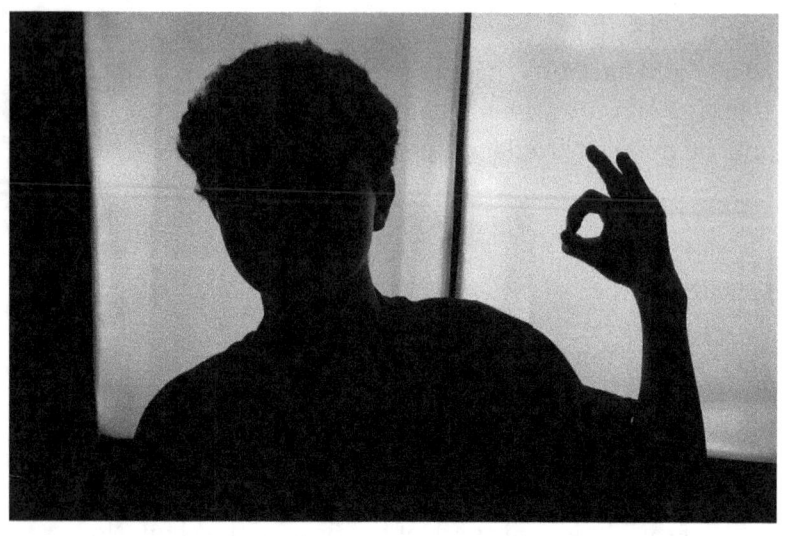

KEGELS

The chances are good that you have heard of this exercise either on television, or saw something on it in a magazine. Women have used Kegel exercises (sometimes called "pelvic floor exercises") for a variety of reasons, including improved sexual performance.

As it turns out, men can benefit from this exercise too. Doing "Kegels" can help improve erections and reduce the likelihood of premature ejaculation. These exercises are also helpful in treating erectile dysfunction. If you are an older man who suffers from urinary leakage, this exercise can also help you reduce those occurrences. In short, if you're a man of any age, Kegel exercises are a worthwhile addition to your day.

In addition to being helpful, Kegel exercises are also easy to do. All you need to do is clench your lower pelvic muscles (these are the same muscles you use to stop your urine stream).

You should hold this clench for a count of five, and then repeat for a total of 10 repetitions according to the WebMD web site. The web site also recommends doing this three times a day. With practice, you should be able to hold the clench for five to 10 seconds and start seeing results in about two to three months. While there are many products available that claim to help with Kegel exercises, there is no need to spend money on them and not a lot of evidence to suggest they work anyway, particularly for men. In fact, several British medical journals have published reports from clinical studies showing that Kegel exercises should be chosen before nerve stimulation (TENS) or other devices.

So, they don't cost anything, are known to be effective, don't cause pain, don't need any kind of equipment and help with a lot of things including achieving better erections and preventing premature ejaculation and urinary incontinence. Why don't they teach this stuff in health class?

Ballooning

Advocates of this exercise claim it can increase penis length as much as three inches, supposedly by reclaiming the shaft of the penis that has sunken into the groin. They also claim it can lead to longer erections, prevent premature ejaculation and help cure erectile dysfunction. Since it doesn't cost anything, and isn't likely to do any damage to your body, it's certainly worth considering.

Here's how to perform the ballooning exercise. This is one exercise you can do with a partner by the way, and since you need to be aroused to do it, might be better off having them help.

1. Become aroused to the point of erection (masturbating if need be).

2. Hold in your ejaculation. This is generally done by placing the hand over the urethral opening, or by squeezing the tip of the penis.

3. Repeat five to six times if you can.

4. During this period, you or your partner should provide some genital massage with or without a lubricant.

5. Some sites also recommend performing Kegel exercises while ballooning in order to increase blood flow to the penis.

The idea behind ballooning is that it makes the spongy tissue of the penis stretch, allowing for more blood saturation in the area that helps maintain erection size and duration.

It may take a few attempts to get the hang of ballooning, and the occasional failure may occur where you do end up ejaculating (obviously not a terrible thing). Still, even if the results are less than you desired, done properly, ballooning should be at least a pleasant exercise.

Many practitioners recommend rubbing your "magic spot." This is the area of the penis that provides the greatest arousal and hardest erection. They also maintain it is different for every man, so it is impossible to say specifically where it is located.

Some suggested places to try include the sides of the shaft, the head of the penis, and the top of the glans (the mushroom like area of the head of the penis right below the topmost point). Two places to avoid are the underside of the glans (the ridge that connects the shaft to the head of the penis, and the frenulum, that small ridge of tissue on the underside of the penis that connects the head to the shaft. These two places can be so sensitive that holding back ejaculation while stimulating them may be impossible.

Proponents of ballooning say that if someone puts in the time and effort to get the hang of the exercise, they can achieve better orgasms, and have better control of those orgasms. Another potential benefit of ballooning is it may lead to "dry" orgasms. These orgasms occur without ejaculation and make it possible (supposedly) for a man to have multiple orgasms.

COMPRESSION

Think of this one as a reverse stretching exercise. It is another way of trying to increase cell growth and can be particularly good at increasing girth. A 2001 study showed that women preferred a thicker penis more than a longer one. So anything that increases your girth will likely help you in the bedroom.

Here's how you do a penis compression exercise:

1. Grasp the base of your penis using an overhand grip. Use a fairly tight, but not choking grip.

2. With your other hand, form an okay symbol and place it below the head of the penis beyond the glans (the bottom end of the head of the penis).

3. Bring both hands together (slowly) squeezing the penis shaft.

4. Carefully bend the shaft back and forth.

Two handed stretch

Another exercise involves grasping the head of the penis with one hand and using the other hand to grasp the base of the shaft, then pulling in opposite directions. Hold this for 10 seconds. Take a short break, then repeat. Try to do this for five minutes a day.

If you've tried exercises, pills, nutrition, and the other stuff covered in this book and it hasn't helped, then perhaps a surgical approach is necessary. This next chapter will provide information on that subject. But first, let's cover devices that might give you some help.

Devices to Improve Size and Performance

There are a number of devices available that claim to help you get a bigger or longer penis. Some of these devices can help, while others won't do much for your penis, but might help your sex life if you don't find them too embarrassing.

We'll take a look at what's on the market and how they're used and how well they work. Some of these seem pretty reasonable, while others call for a leap of faith on the user's part. Let's start with devices to make the penis bigger.

The lack of research on the effectiveness of these devices is a constant in this book. While there is a lot of information on plastic surgery for injury reconstruction and for other types of cosmetic surgery, this particular area has not drawn much interest from researchers or medical specialists, probably because of a societal stigma on the subject.

PENIS ENLARGERS – PENIS PUMPS

The first type of penis enlarger is the penis pump, or, more properly, vacuum constriction device. These tools can be simple and inexpensive or technologically advanced and pricey. They work on the principle of using suction to pull more blood into the penis and make it bigger. (Yes, I know "suction" usually does make the penis bigger, but this does it differently than a bout of oral stimulation.)

The good news is that penis pumps can actually provide some help. Unfortunately, the help is on more of a temporary basis. Even more important, if the user overdoes it, he can seriously hurt himself. There is not a lot of data on whether or not there may be any long term effects of using a penis pump on a daily basis.

To use a penis pump, the open end is placed over the shaft and against the groin, making sure to create a good seal. Often, a water soluble jelly is applied to the ring first. The user then either pumps the hand pump or activates the device if using an automated unit.

The vacuum causes the entire penis to both lengthen and thicken slowly. You may also notice your penis picking up a bluish tinge or feeling a bit cold. This is not unusual or anything to be worried about. Using a penis pump will also cause a slightly uncomfortable sensation that some may find a little bit painful even when the device is used properly. This is part of the cost to its benefits. Speaking of cost, penis pumps can cost anywhere from $20 or less to several hundred dollars. It can take as long as 10 to 20 minutes before you achieve a full erection using one. If you have trouble maintaining a good seal, try shaving around the pubic area to improve the seal.

They are generally considered safe, but if you decide to try one, make sure it has a quick release mechanism, because there have been reports of these devices being hard to remove without one.

You may experience some bruising around the area where the pump chamber meets the groin, but this is usually not painful. The bruises disappear after a few days. Another consideration is that the erection a penis pump produces isn't exactly an equal to one achieved naturally both in appearance and results. Ejaculation will more than likely be reduced and less forceful because of the constriction at the shaft of the penis. This last issue is usually the result of a constriction band or cock ring used after the penis is erect (cock rings are covered in a few paragraphs).

There are some risks to using a penis pump. If you take blood thinners or have sickle cell anemia or another blood disorder that affects bleeding or blood clotting, using one can cause increased bleeding.

Still, if you're not getting anywhere in trying to get an erection, a penis pump and cock ring (covered next) will certainly improve your situation.

PENIS PUMPS THAT USE WATER

So far, the penis pumps we've been discussing have worked under the principle of creating a vacuum over the penis in order to draw blood into the penis shaft. These pumps use a combination of air and water to do the same. The supposed advantage is that because water can't be compressed to any measurable degree, it provides an advantage over air, which can lead to uneven results (strange bulges).

The manufacturers usually claim that only about 15 to 20 minutes of use will result in a larger penis. They also say the device should be used regularly for the best results.

While these devices can be used without water, the manufacturers recommend using them in the bath or shower for best results. They are a little more complex than your basic penis pump, and as a result are more expensive. At the low end, they can cost above $100. At the high end, they can cost well over $200.

Manufacturers claim these types of penis pumps can produce long lasting and superior results.

CHARTHAM METHOD

There is a variation on the basic penis pump method that was created by a medical doctor (Robert Chartham, a pseudonym of Ronald Sydney Seth, a British writer). This is more in depth than just using a penis pump and its purpose is to help promote a bigger penis and not just temporarily. There are several additional steps to this method beginning with giving your penis a deep massage with a cream lotion loosen up the fibers of the penis.

Next, place the penis pump over the flaccid penis. Note, it is important to do this with a flaccid penis and not an erect one. If your penis massage causes an erection, then you'll need to wait until it subsides. (Most men think about baseball to accomplish this, but others find visualizing an ex or their grandparents having sex to also work.)

Make sure you have a good seal against the groin and begin pumping. Take your time and don't stop just because you have the beginnings of an erection. Once you are erect, a few more pumps will be necessary.

Once you've gotten to maximum size, let air into the pump quickly (your pump should have a quick release valve) and then wait for your erection to subside. You can insert it into a container of cold water if you want to speed up the process.

Once your penis has returned to its flaccid state, grasp the base of the shaft and slowly, but firmly give several tugs. Once completed, then repeat the whole process.

There was a medical study in the 1970s that reported positive results with this method. Participants did show gains of about an inch to an inch and a half in length and from a half inch to an inch in girth.

Unfortunately, no follow up research was ever performed, in part because of the prevailing opinion in the medical community that exercises could not improve penis size.

COCK RINGS

The proper name for these aids is "Penoscrotal" rings, but few people refer to them that way. Cock rings don't do anything to permanently enhance a penis, but they do work reasonably well on a temporary basis.

These elastic rings fit over the shaft of the penis and are placed all the way at the bottom of the shaft. They constrict the penis there, forcing more blood into the shaft and head above the cock ring and also preventing blood from leaving the penis. They can work particularly well with a penis pump. After using the pump to enlarge the penis, the cock ring will help maintain the effects of the pump. They can also help you to maintain an erection.

Cock rings are inexpensive (often less than $10, and are sometimes even given away with other purchases) and come in a variety of shapes and designs ranging from the simple to the wacky. You can even find versions that can accept a small "bullet" vibrator for even more pleasure (at least that's the advertising claim).

The use of these erection aids comes with one word of warning though. It is a bad idea to wear one for a half hour or more because constricting the blood flow to the penis can eventually be harmful.

Cock rings are generally made of some kind of stretchy material, but it is possible to find examples made of metal. Users need to very careful if using one of these because of the swelling that occurs because of the blood they trap in the penis. Cock rings that can stretch are easier to remove than ones that can't. If you were unable to remove a metal cock ring, you could end up seriously hurting yourself.

Also, there is a technique called "Clamping," that involves the use of a cock ring along with "edging." Edging is a technique where you masturbate close to ejaculation but stop before going over the edge. Edging is a technique some people use to try to make their penis bigger, but combining it with a cock ring can be very dangerous. In a worst case scenario, it can lead to amputation.

PENIS CAGES

This is a variation on the cock ring. The device is a plastic or latex cage that stretches over the shaft of the penis. Some versions also have a ring that stretches over the testes too. The advantages to the cage approach is that it supports the shaft of the penis better in addition to adding the constriction to firm up your member. You can also find versions that include a bullet vibrator designed to "tickle her fancy," in just the right spot.

These appliances can be helpful since they constrict more of the penis and often have a testicular loop, which also helps improve your erection. It's a good idea to use some lubrication on the inside of the penis cage to make it easier to get on and off. Some versions will encompass the entire shaft and head, while others leave the head of the penis free for a more enjoyable sensation.

If you need immediate improvement and aren't worried about appearances, then a penis extender may be the answer you are looking for. These are sort of an imitation penis that fits over yours providing greater length and girth. Some even are designed to let the head of your penis extend out the end of the device so you can enjoy more of the sexual sensations. These versions usually do more to thicken your member rather than lengthen it. The good news is that when surveyed, a majority of women said girth made a bigger difference than length, so this might be an option worth considering.

There's no real physical risk to using one of these unless you leave them on too long (30 minutes or mroe) and they come in all sorts of shapes and sizes. Some attach to the end of your member, while others are sleeve like devices that fit over the entire shaft. There are even battery powered versions that vibrate during use.

Prices for these devices range from less than $10 to $30, $40, or more.

PENIS EXTENDERS (FOR STRETCHING THE PENIS)

You can also find devices designed to stretch your penis with the idea of making it longer over time. The principle behind the penis stretcher is that regular use causes microscopic tears in the shaft of the penis causing gaps in the tissue, which the body then fills. It can take several months to a year for the process to work.

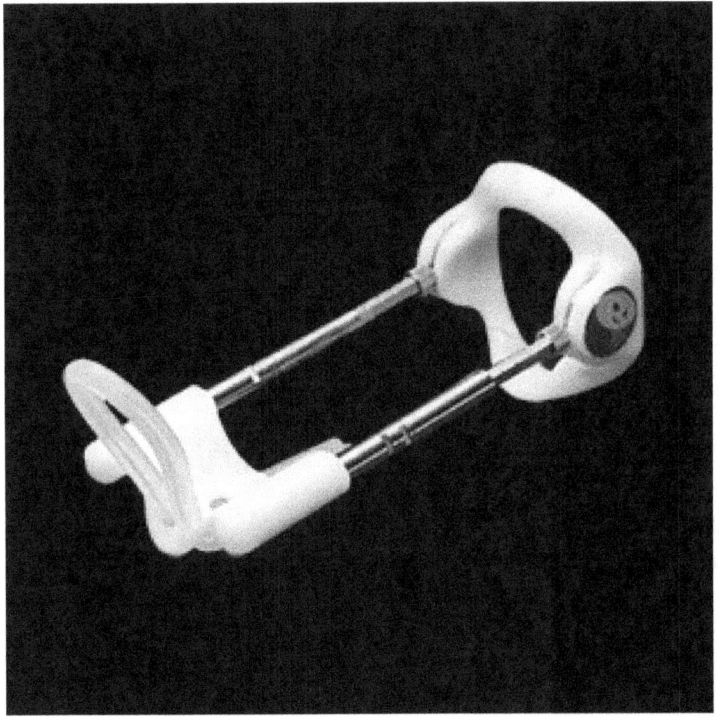

These are more expensive than the penis extenders mentioned earlier, but they need to be better made and more durable because they are worn for longer periods of time and have to maintain tension to keep the penis stretched. Advertisers claim that with proper use, wearers can gain an inch or more of length.

It is important to follow instructions carefully with these devices because improper use can cause pain and injury.

There is some scientific research to support the validity of this treatment. Researchers at the University of Turin in Italy studied the results of surgical and non surgical approaches to penis enlargement. They found that wearing the device for an appropriate period of time (about four hours a day for four to six months) did achieve positive results.

A study conducted by Jørn Ege Siana, MD, a Danish plastic surgeon and Urologist (a specialist in problems affecting the male genitalia) was presented to International Interdisciplinary Symposium on Genitourinary Reconstructive Surgery in April 1998.

In that study, 18 test subjects (ages 23 to 47), with normal erectile function, used a penis traction device for 26 weeks for a total of 1,100 hours. Medical personnel also checked them every two weeks.

By the end of the study, the participants had gained an average of 29 percent greater length. There were no complications reported and every participant was shown to have increased in length.

Another study that year consisting of 37 adults (22 to 60 years old) showed similar results. The studies appear to have shown the most important thing is total hours of traction. It didn't matter whether it was more hours over a shorter period of time or fewer hours over a longer period of time. Both studies used type 1 medical devices. This means a medical body has actually certified the devices to be safe and to do what they are supposed to do.

This is important because to be effective devices need to be able to maintain precise and consistent traction. They also have to be comfortable to wear (obviously).

Now, before you start dangling weights off you best buddy, keep a couple of things in mind. First of all, 54 people are not much of a sample size. Even more importantly, there doesn't seem to have been any follow up information available. A natural question is did they keep their added length or did their penises shrink after a period of time?

So if you really want to extend the length of your penis, this approach seems to be one practice that could really make a difference. Just keep in mind that you will be earning that extension through a sustained, uncomfortable effort.

If you are going to give this a try, look for one that will be comfortable enough to wear underneath your clothing. Test it while standing, sitting, and walking, plus any other movements you expect to go through during the course of a normal day.

HANGING WEIGHTS

No I'm not joking. You can actually buy devices that make it possible for you hang weights off your penis to stretch it. Users will suspend as much as 10 pounds or more off their member and let them hang for a specific period of time. Historical research shows this may be the oldest version of man's efforts at penis enlargement.

Obviously, the user needs to be careful, since the possibility of actually injuring you penis is high. (Something I would have to be to even consider this approach.)

If you are going to try something like this, make sure you follow the directions carefully and start out with minimal weight and gradually increase the weight your best buddy is carrying safely.

The logic behind this approach is found in the efforts of those cultures that deliberately stretch a part of their body (usually lips, or necks). From a medical standpoint, "continuous traction" on the tissues of the penis causes cellular multiplication. This results in permanent tissue expansion. Unfortunately there really isn't a lot of research on this method, in part because it is a very difficult thing to test. Still, there is some evidence for some small improvement via this method when it comes to increasing length, but not girth. If you decide you want to try stretching via hanging weights, understand it will be uncomfortable, will take a lot of dedication, and time, and, if you are not careful, injury or permanent damage. You should talk to a doctor if planning on beginning such a program.

Another problem with the lack of research in this area is that it is hard to know how much weight to use, how long it should be used, and how diligent the patient must be.

CHAPTER 5: BASIC HEALTH AND YOUR PENIS

Your health can definitely affect your penis whether it be your ability to achieve and maintain an erection, or affect the apparent size of it.

Because this is a complex issue, this chapter will cover basic health issues that apply to all ages, then look at specific age based complications. Obviously, a 65 year old man and a 20 year old man are going to have different issues affecting their size and performance. Let's get started.

The web site Livestrong.com sites information from the National Heart, Lung and Blood Institute, saying risk factors for erectile dysfunction include high blood pressure, high cholesterol levels, smoking, obesity, diabetes and unhealthy diet.

While it isn't any fun to hear, improving your diet and physical condition can do a lot to help with impaired erectile function and apparent size. Quitting smoking can also help. Too much alcohol can also inhibit erections, so cutting back on booze when you are expecting intercourse can also help.

Unfortunately, many health concerns that arise from poor health and nutrition, also lead to sexual performance problems. Even if the problems (blood pressure, type II diabetes, and others) don't directly cause problems, the medications used to treat these problems often will.

Aging also leads to its share of problems that can lead to decreased performance too. Testosterone levels can decrease, as can levels of nitric oxide, which plays an important role in getting and maintaining an erection.

Atherosclerosis, a narrowing and hardening of the arteries associated with heart disease can also lead to erectile dysfunction because of reduced blood flow to various parts of the body including the penis.

Go for a walk

You don't need to be an Olympic athlete to enjoy good sexual health. If you are having issues though, adding a walk to your daily routine can help more than you might think. Ideally, you should walk about two miles a day according to a study a few years back.

This doesn't mean you should run right out and start walking two miles if you're not up to it. Even some additional physical activity will make a difference and the more you do, the greater the results.

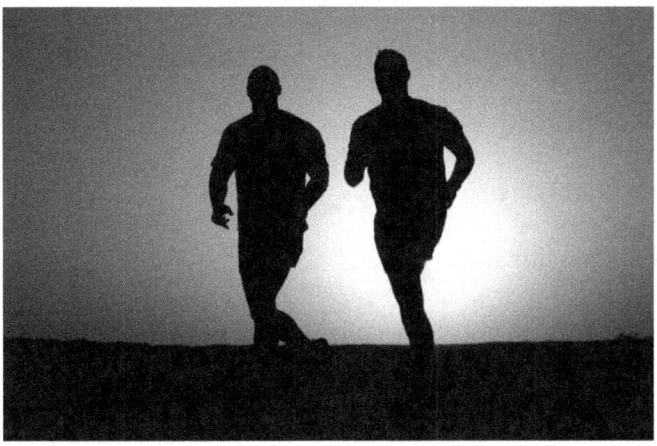

GOOD NUTRITION

Certain foods can affect your ability to get and maintain an erection. Some can help and some can hurt. A 2010 study showed the Mediterranean diet (a diet high in fruits, vegetables, nuts, seeds, and olive oil) were associated with recovery from erectile dysfunction, according to the Journal of Sexual Medicine.

If you want to try eating better to improve your sex life, the following foods can help:

- Fish

- Deeply colored fruits and vegetables

- Nitric oxide producing compounds

- Red wine

- Lean meats

- Pistachios

- Watermelon

Obviously, these foods won't break the bank and certainly offer something for most palates. If you also need to lose weight, these can help too.

On the other hand, low carb diets can be part of the problem, so if you are one of those diets, it may be part of the problem.

One thing to also consider is that erectile dysfunction can also be a precursor to heart disease. This is another reason why you should consult with your doctor.

FOODS TO AVOID

Foods that are high in fat aren't good for your heart or your blood vessels. Seeing as blood flow to the penis is the foundation of an erection, anything that reduces blood flow affects size and erection.

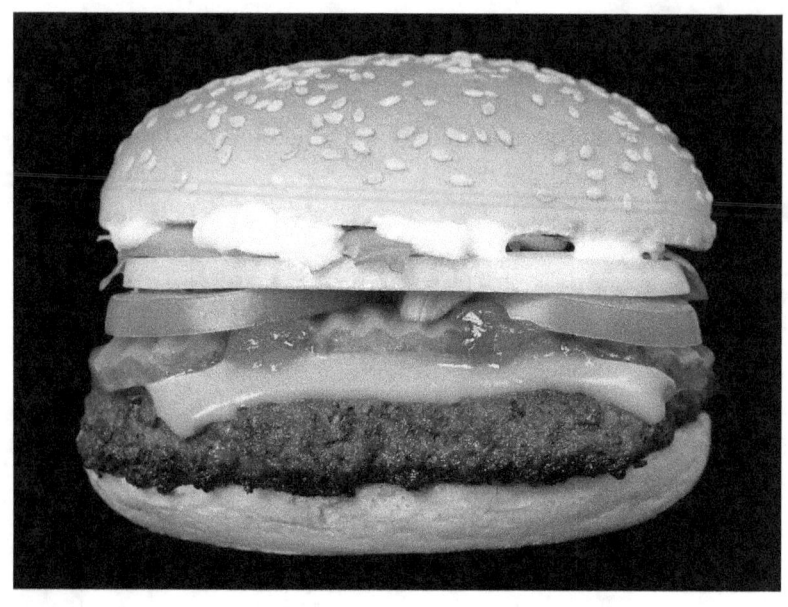

WEIGHT

If you're overweight it will affect your apparent penis size and performance. I know this is frustrating to hear. I'm fat myself, and I see how it affects me. I don't think it's much of a stretch to think it may affect you the same way.

As mentioned earlier, the fatter you are, the more apparent length you lose. I say "apparent" because you aren't actually losing anything. It's just that the shaft of the penis sinks into the fat in the groin. You can lose an inch or more this way.

Being overweight also costs you energy and self confidence, two things that can also impact your sex life. It isn't so much that being heavier affects your bedroom efforts, it is the things that tend to accompany the excess weight that cause the problems. Exercise can help with blood flow to the groin and penis, which will help you. This will be covered later in this book.

Conditions such as high cholesterol, high blood pressure, or insulin resistance can either affect your ability to get and maintain an erection, or the drugs your doctor prescribes to deal with these issues can be the cause. There are a lot of drugs that can reduce your libido, and or your ability to get and maintain an erection.

Losing weight can certainly help too. Even dropping 10 pounds can make a difference. Another thing that can weaken your ability to get and maintain an erection is tight pants. Wearing looser fitting trousers or sweats may help. If you suspect your meds are hampering your love life talk to your doctor. They may be able to change or adjust your prescription(s) to help.

As a general rule of thumb, for every 35 pounds of excess weight a man loses, his penis gains an inch of length.

DIABETES PREVENTION OR REVERSAL

Erectile dysfunction tends to show up 10 to 15 years earlier in men with diabetes than those who don't suffer from this problem. If you have type I diabetes, there isn't much changing your diet or lifestyle can do. Those suffering from type II diabetes on the other hand can do quite a bit. Losing weight and being careful about your diet can reverse type II diabetes, particularly if you are in the pre-insulin phase of the affliction.

PHYSICAL OR PSYCHOLOGICAL?

Erectile dysfunction can be caused by physical or psychological issues, but usually has a physical origin.

Generally, if it becomes a problem gradually over time, you can figure a physical issue is more likely the cause. On the other hand, if it seems to become a problem overnight, then a psychological issue may be the cause. Depression for example can be a cause of erectile dysfunction.

HEALTH PROBLEMS

If you are being treated for prostate cancer, then your chances of developing erectile dysfunction increase, getting worse as you get older. The likelihood of your treatment causing this problem is greater if your cancer has been treated surgically than if you were treated with radiation.

Chapter 6: Surgical and other Medical Approaches

Drastic times call for drastic measures. If you've tried the other solutions in this book and are willing to consider everything the medical profession has to offer, then perhaps surgery will be your answer.

Keep in mind that penis enlargement surgery is usually not covered by insurance since it is considered cosmetic in nature. While there are several surgical options available, the simplest and easiest answer is liposuction to remove excess fat from the groin area (remember those inches that sink into the fat?).

If you want something more significant, then there are several different procedures that involving grafting skin from other parts of the body to the penis. In truth, these seldom provide all that much improvement and when they do, it's usually only seen in the flaccid penis, not during an erection.

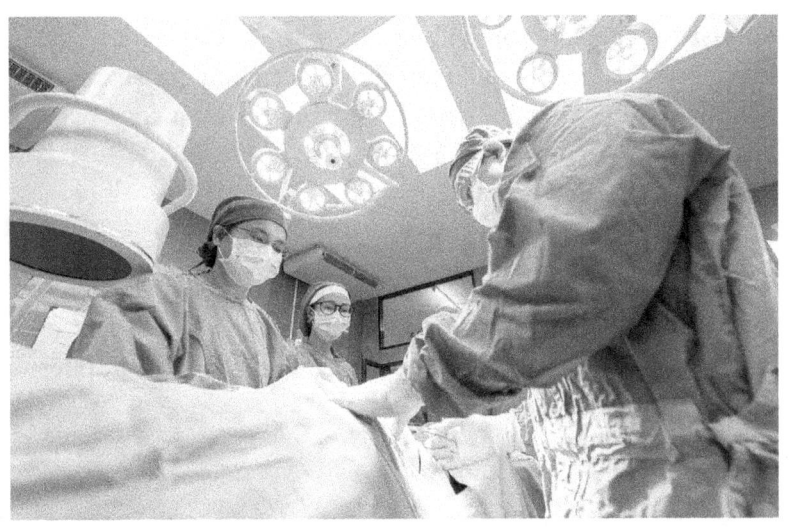

SURGERY FOR PENIS ENLARGEMENT

If you are a woman who wants bigger breasts, there is a thriving area of medicine devoted just to make that a reality for you. Sadly, no such option exists for men.

While there are a couple of surgical options for men who want a larger penis, these approaches are of limited results. One such approach involves severing a ligament that attaches the penis to the pelvic bone. This might get you almost an inch, but you will also have to wear weights suspended from your penis for hours each day for six months to prevent the ligament from reattaching. This surgery can cost anywhere from $3,500 to more than $9,000.

Another possible surgery works only for men whose scrotum attaches high up on the penis. In this case the scrotum is partially disconnected from the shaft increasing the apparent length.

If you want a thicker penis, there are a couple of questionable approaches that involve either tissue grafting or implanting fat or silicone.

There is some concern about these approaches. The American Urologic Association has said they have not been shown to be "safe or effective." There are no studies or clinical trials showing their effectiveness either.

PENUMA

There is a new surgical approach to penis enlargement that does show some promise. It is known as "Penuma" and was pioneered by a Beverly Hills urologist. It involves surgically implanting a silicone sheath inside the penis, making the penis longer and thicker. Dr. James Elist, the inventor, is currently the only doctor approved by the FDA to perform Penuma surgery. The implant sheath itself has not been FDA approved, but it has been cleared by the FDA to be used commercially.

The surgery costs about $13,000 and men receiving the implant must abstain from sex for six weeks. You must be circumcised for this surgery, but Dr. Elist will do that for you if you aren't. So far the results have averaged about two to two and a half inches improvement from the implant surgery, but the doctor says those numbers will increase almost 100 percent as its time in the patient increases.
QWTWTHHHWWWTT

Oh yes, it comes in three sizes: "Large (L)," "Extra Large (XL)," and "Double Extra Large (XXL). This is because nobody wants a "small" or a "medium" jokes the inventor, who as of January 2016 had implanted more than 1,300 of the sheaths.

SURGERY FOR ERECTILE DYSFUNCTION

While there are few if any surgical solutions for someone who feels their penis needs to be bigger, there are some for those suffering from erectile dysfunction.

The problem with surgery for erectile dysfunction is it invasive, and as with any surgery, incurs risks of infection. Because of that, medical practitioners try to work with non-invasive and minimally invasive procedures before turning to surgical answers.

Most commonly, doctors either try to repair blood vessels in the penis that have been damaged by diabetes or implants featuring rods that provide the erection.

BLOOD VESSEL REPAIR

In cases where injury has damaged a blood vessel in the penis resulting in erectile dysfunction, surgery is becoming an option. In this surgery, which is not recommended for people whose erective dysfunction is from high blood pressure or diabetes, the surgeon grafts a blood vessel from one part of the body and implants it into the penis.

Unfortunately, this surgery tends to be expensive. It's also technically difficult, and there's not a lot of evidence to say it works either. Unless you are a young man who suffered a damaged blood vessel in the penis due to injury, it's not worth considering. And if you are a young man who suffered a damaged blood vessel in the penis due to injury, its success rate is poor.

IMPLANTS

Penis implants have been used for quite a while now and have been pretty successful at helping men with erectile dysfunction. Even better, the technology has been improving over the years.

In simple terms, penile implants are rods that are surgically inserted into the penis. They can be inflatable or malleable (molded by hand). The malleable version features a single rod, while the inflatable rod uses two rods. The advantage to the inflatable system is it also improves length and thickness.

These devices can last from a decade to 25 years or more. The more a man uses them, the more likely the probability of something going wrong.

The inflatables come with a pump that is positioned by the scrotum (either side is fine), and inside the scrotum out of view. The user pumps it to inflate the implant, and once finished, deflates it. Penile implants have been implanted in men as old as 90 years old.

Surgery usually requires a small incision. In some versions the incision is made in the scrotum, in others, it is made in the lower abdomen. It usually takes about 20 minutes and is handled as an outpatient procedure for most patients. Recovery time takes about two to three weeks for full recovery and you can expect to miss two to three days from work.

There have been occasional problems with implants including inflating on their own, the pump shifting, and the device breaking.

TESTOSTERONE GELS

Testosterone gels can also be helpful with erectile dysfunction and may also add a little bit to penis size. Users apply the gel to their shoulder or shoulders. The gel may need a few days or longer to show any effects, and it can be used with erectile dysfunction drugs too. Low testosterone doesn't necessarily cause erectile dysfunction, but if you suffer from it, then a testosterone substitute can help. These are prescription drugs, so you'll need to consult with a doctor to get a prescription for one.

PRIAPUS SHOT

This is a relatively new medical option. It is a more complicated procedure than the shots described earlier in this book, which is why it is in this section rather than the section on drugs. Another reason is that it doesn't really involve actual drugs per se.

The treatment involves harvesting the patient's blood, which is then spun in a centrifuge. The result is platelet rich plasma. While platelets are the body's tool for stopping bleeding, they also help growth.

The first thing that happens is the penis is numbed, then the doctor injects the plasma into the patient's penis in five different spots.

For the next month or two, the man uses a penis pump for 10 minutes each day. The treatment is said to increase penis size by 10 to 20 percent and the results are supposed to be permanent. The one time treatment (one treatment is "usually" enough) costs about $2,500.

It is a pretty new treatment and the results are mostly anecdotal. Recipients have said the Priapus shot works well, and they usually have no regrets about having had the treatment. There is little if any "hard" evidence of its effectiveness as of yet.

There is also a version of this treatment for women that supposedly result in better and more frequent orgasms.

One last benefit of this approach is that since the patient's own blood is used, there is pretty much no chance of rejection or adverse reaction.

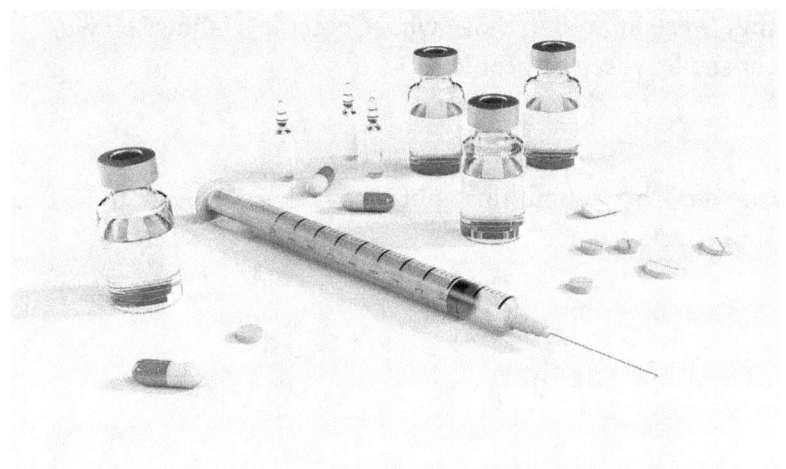

ELECTRIC SHOCK TREATMENT

A not yet approved treatment for erectile dysfunction uses a form of electric shock. It is called "low intensity shock wave treatment" and it works by increasing blood flow to the penis.

So far it has mainly been tested on animals whose "equipment" operates in a manner similar to that of human beings. There have been some studies on its effects on human subjects with varied results. There were a number of positive results reported by the participants, but it seemed they were limited to those whose erectile dysfunction was caused by vascular problems.

One nice thing about this approach is there appears to be few side effects from it.

STEM CELL THERAPY

Another possible therapy for erectile dysfunction is via stem cell treatment. While the initial results have been promising, research into this treatment form is still in its early stages. There are some early phase clinical trials underway. There is also research ongoing looking into using bone marrow cells for erectile dysfunction treatment.

OTHER TREATMENTS

A systematic review of existing and prospective erectile dysfunction treatments published in the June 2016 Arab Journal of Urology, also discussed other potential treatments. These included the following:

- Vibratory stimulation – use of a vibration device to stimulate the nerves. Right now the technology is awaiting controlled clinical trials.

- Impulsive magnetic field therapy – this approach can enhance blood circulation. It is also in the very early stages and a fairly long time away.

- Tissue engineering – this is probably the most futuristic idea we've looked at so far, and is a long ways away. It may someday be possible to utilize them for a biological substitute to a penile prosthesis.

- Nanotechnology – this is also pretty futuristic, although studies have been made of it use on rat penises. There are currently no human trials on the horizon. Researchers are optimistic that this technology could revolutionize erectile dysfunction treatment.

Conclusion

Thank for making it through to the end of *Penis Enlargement Options: Surgery, Stretchers, Pumps, Clamps, Pills, Exercise, and More!* Let's hope it was informative and able to provide you with all of the tools you need to achieve your goals whatever it may be.

The next step is to consult with your physician or sexual health medical professional, to see what their views on this are. As tempting as it may be to start popping all sorts of over the counter supplements and trying different devices, if you are suffering from any number of medical problems (such as high blood pressure or diabetes), unrestrained use of some of these items can be harmful.

Some things, such as the exercises listed in this book, improving your diet, and starting a weight loss program are less risky, but weight loss measures can be potentially risky if you try diet pills or extreme diet approaches.

Here's a list of things you start with right away:

- Change your diet to include better nutrients (including the ones discussed in the chapter on nutrition and health.

- Wear clothing that is loose in the crotch.

- Start going for walks (if you have health problems or are an older man, you may wish to check with your doctor first).

- Try a cock ring.

- Consider a penis pump.

- Start doing exercises such as Kegels, Jengling, and the others covered in the section on exercise (Chapter 4).

- Take a zinc supplement

- Try Horney Goat Weed (Amazon Link)

- Try Mr. Thick (Amazon Link)

Trim the hedges. Trimming your pubic hair will make your penis look bigger. You don't have to shave completely either, just shorten them. This is something your partner will probably really appreciate if oral sex is part of your routine anyway.

Dealing with either erectile dysfunction or a penis that you feel is too small, are both challenges for a man. Either of these situations can affect your self confidence and also add stress to a relationship.

You can look at the idea in this book as covering the short term, mid term and long term and plan accordingly. Perhaps one or two of the short term solutions can help improve your circumstances while you employ the longer term methods to effect more permanent results.

If you are in a relationship, think about confiding in that person. Their help can be important, especially for several of the techniques discussed in these pages.

Finally, if you found this book useful in any way, a review on Amazon is always appreciated!